get well

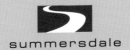
summersdale

To: *Mary*

From: *Ellie .*

GET WELL

Summersdale Publishers Ltd
46 West Street
Chichester
West Sussex
PO19 1RP
UK

www.summersdale.com

Printed and bound by Tien Wah Press, Singapore

ISBN: 978-1-84024-764-0

Substantial discounts on bulk quantities of Summersdale books are available to corporations, professional associations and other organisations. For details telephone Summersdale Publishers on (+44-1243-771107), fax (+44-1243-786300) or email (nicky@summersdale.com).

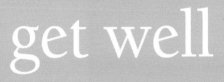

get well

Poppy Bell

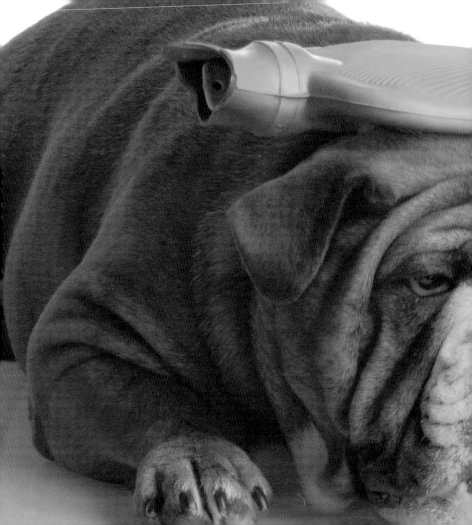

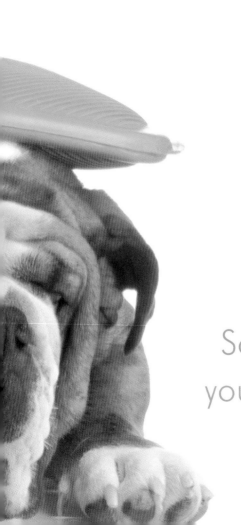

Sorry to hear
you're not well.

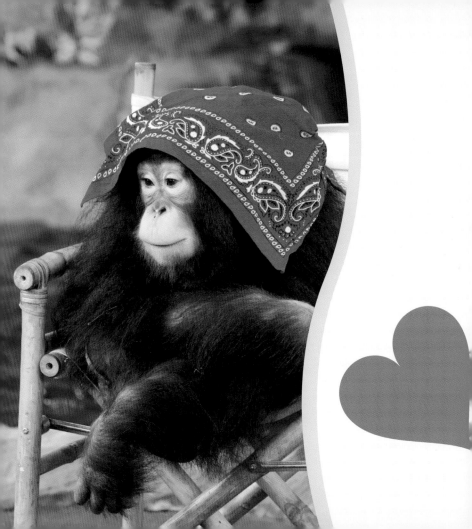

It's hard to keep going when you're feeling fragile...

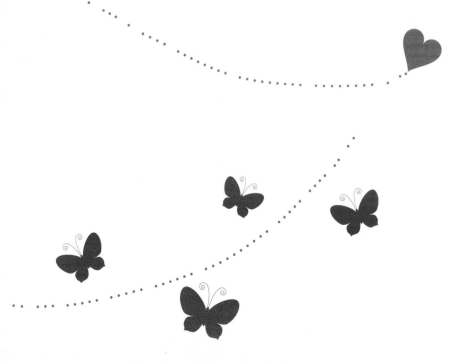

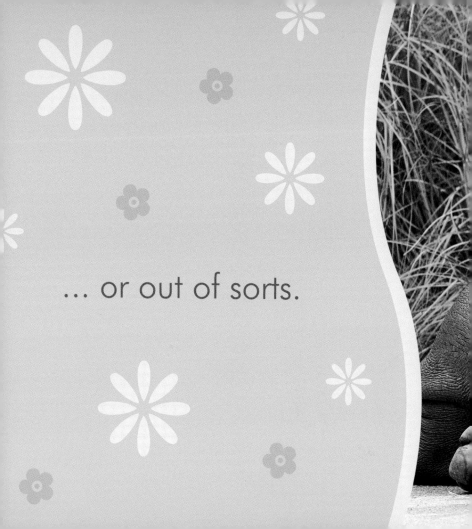

... or out of sorts.

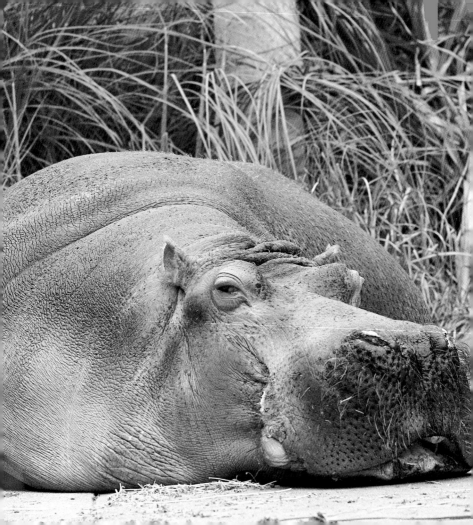

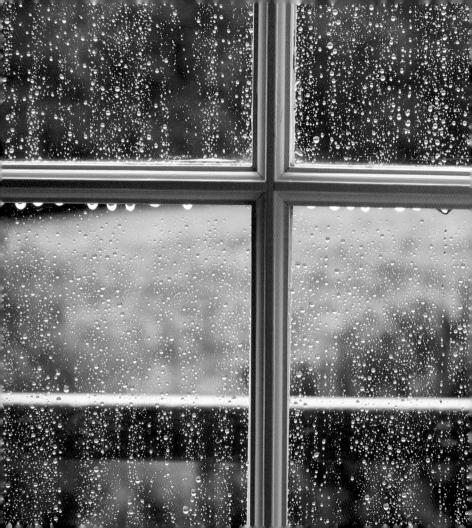

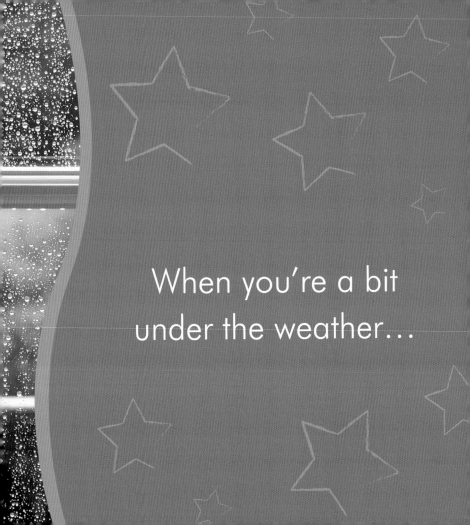

When you're a bit
under the weather...

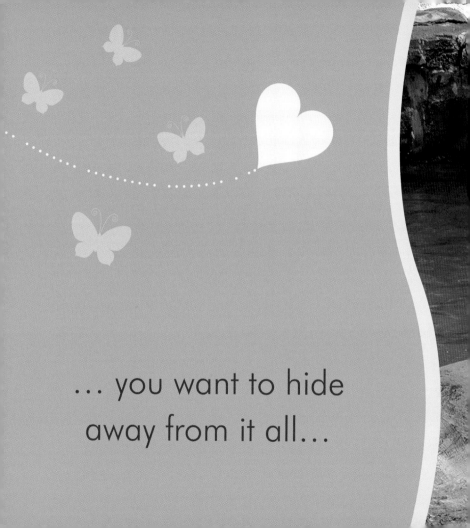

... you want to hide
away from it all...

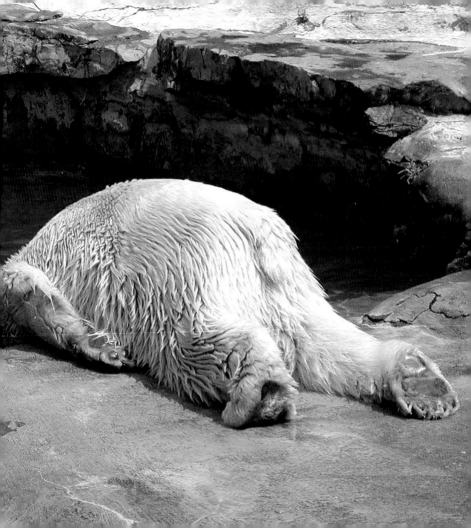

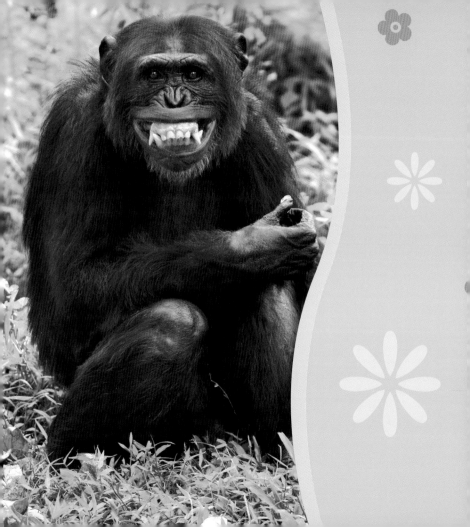

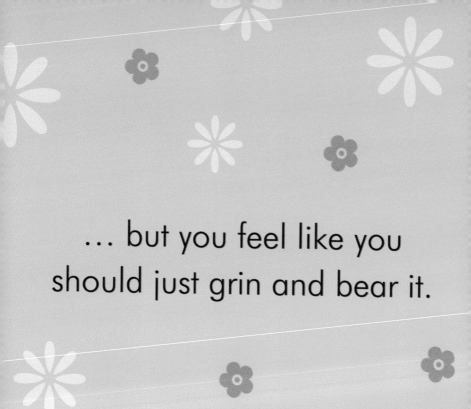

... but you feel like you should just grin and bear it.

At times like
these, you need
to take it easy...

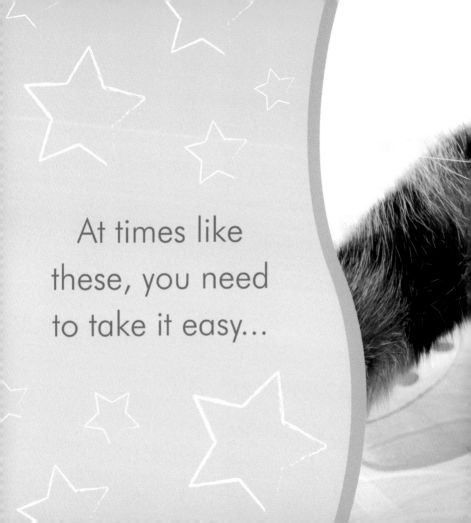

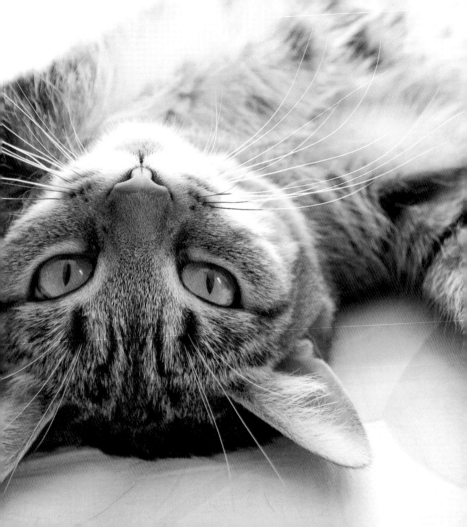

... so put your feet up...

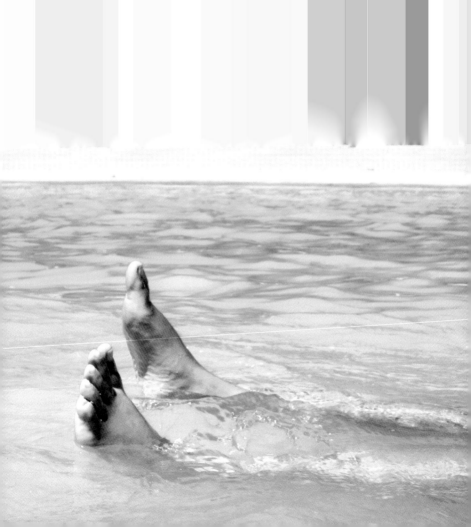

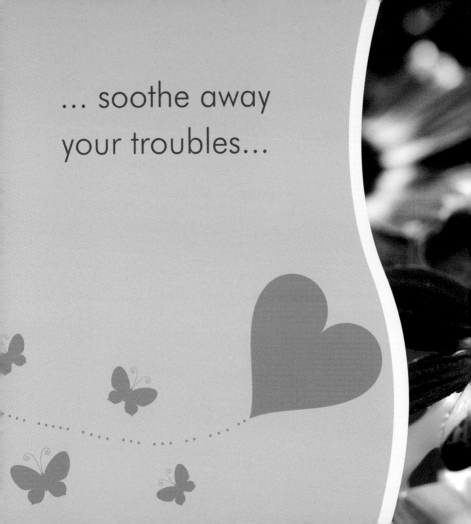

... soothe away
your troubles...

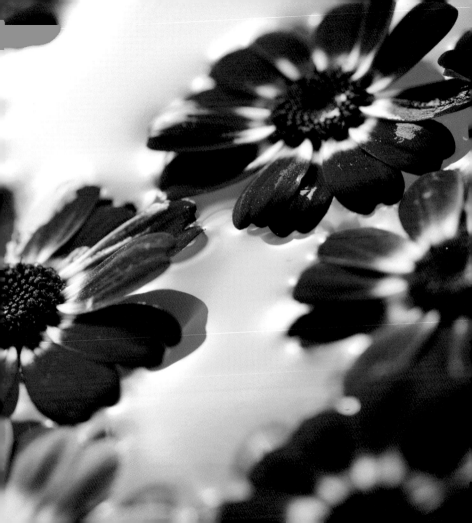

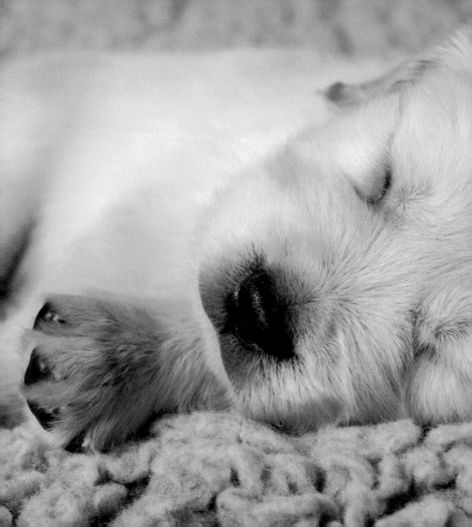

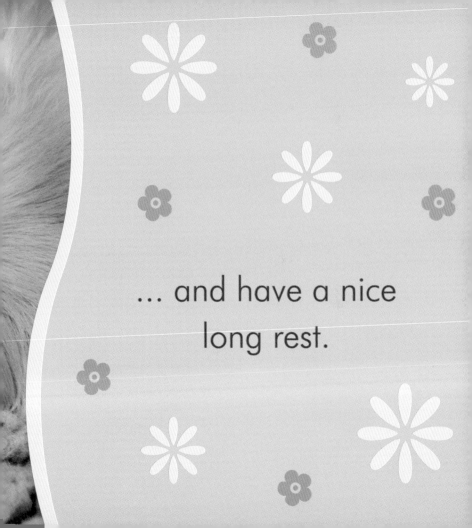

... and have a nice
long rest.

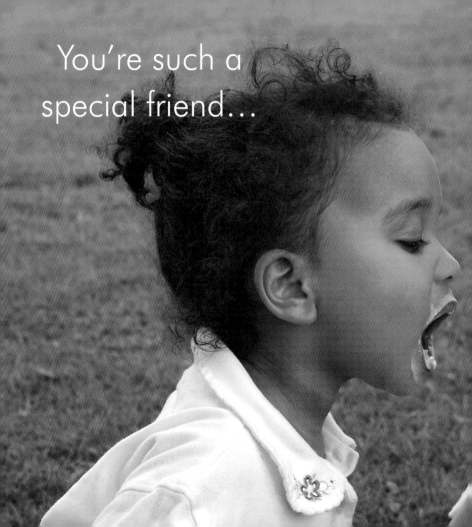

You're such a
special friend...

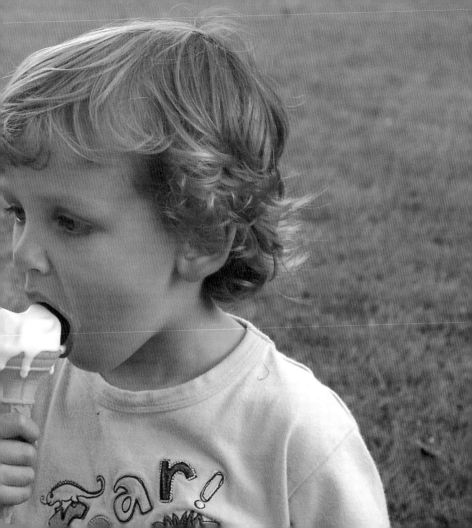

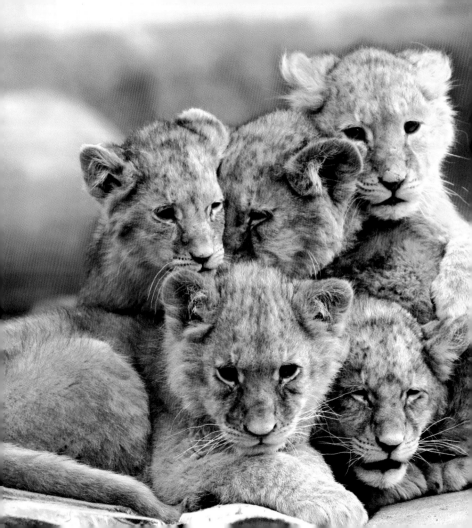

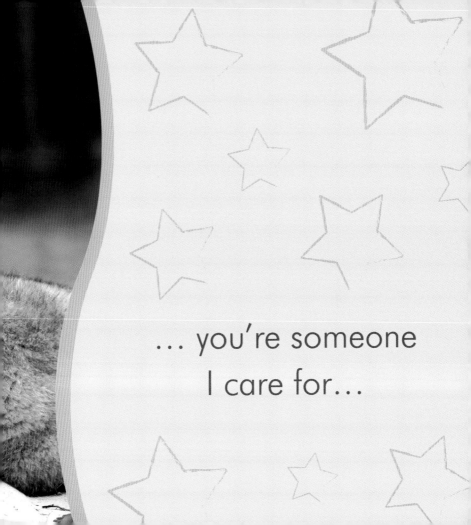

... you're someone
I care for...

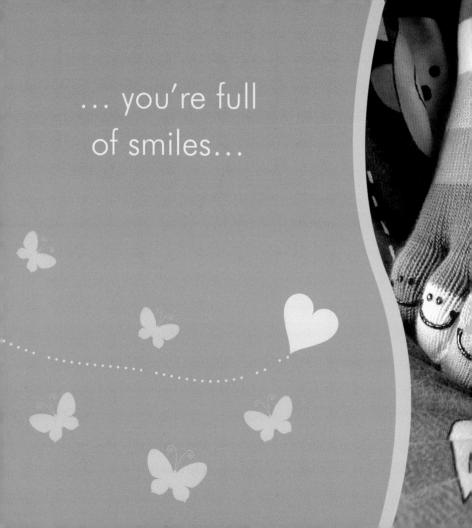

... you're full
of smiles...

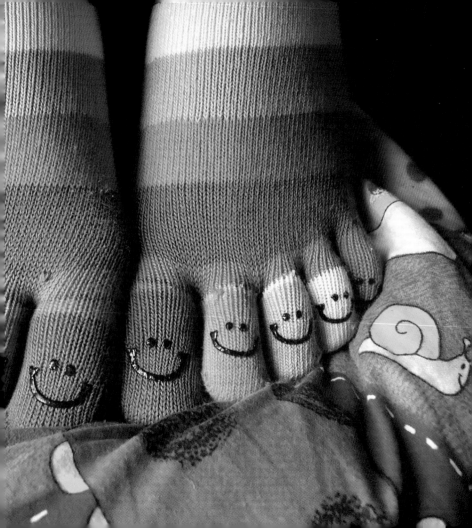

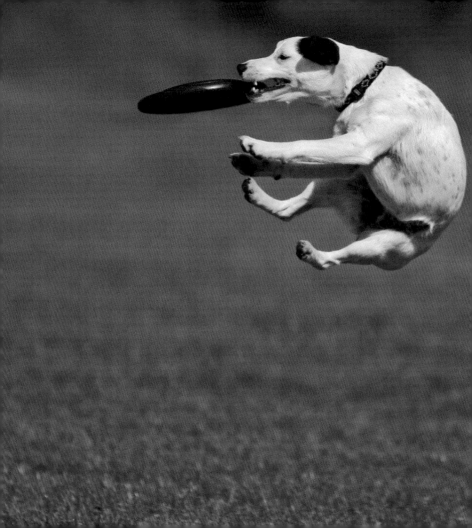

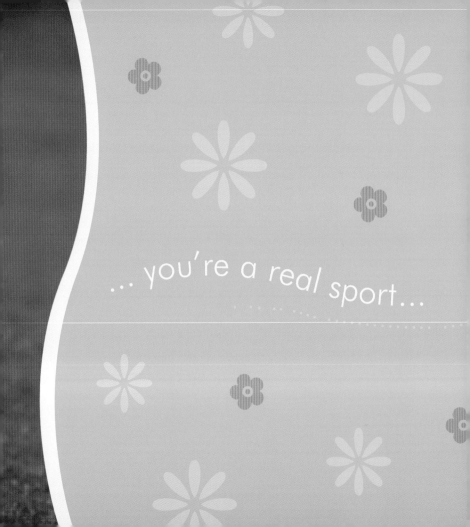

... you're a real sport...

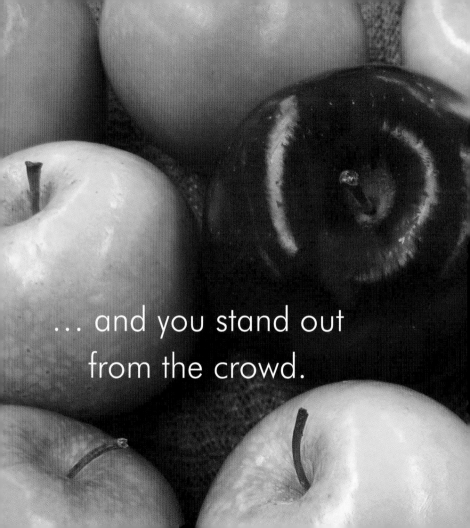

... and you stand out from the crowd.

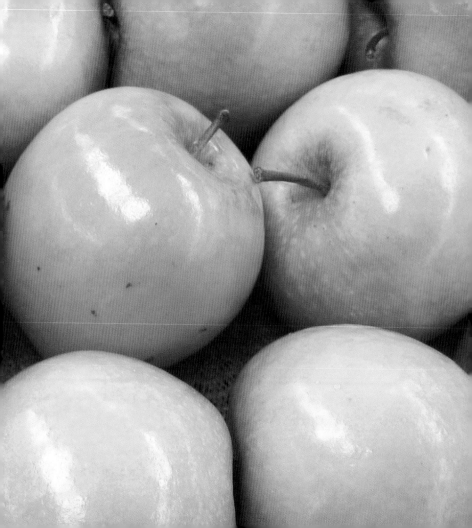

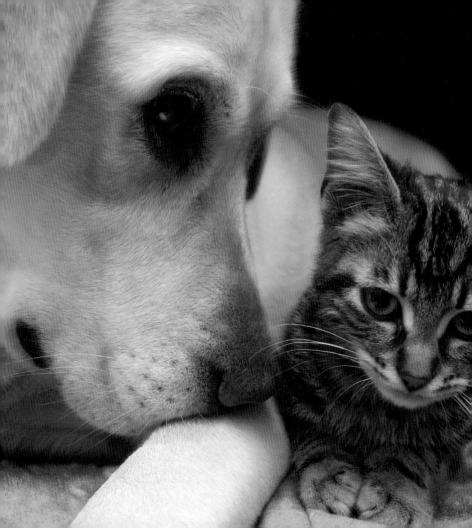

We're here to help.

Now it's time to take care
of yourself – you deserve it!

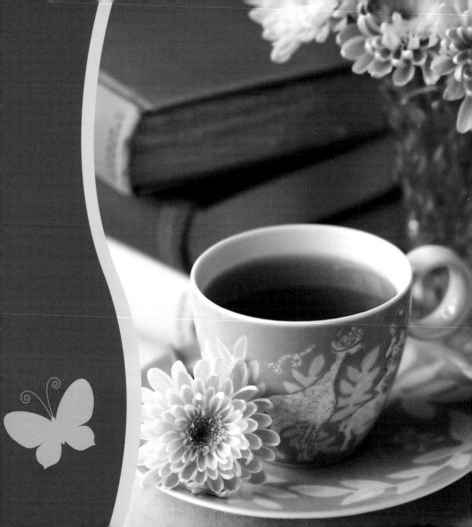

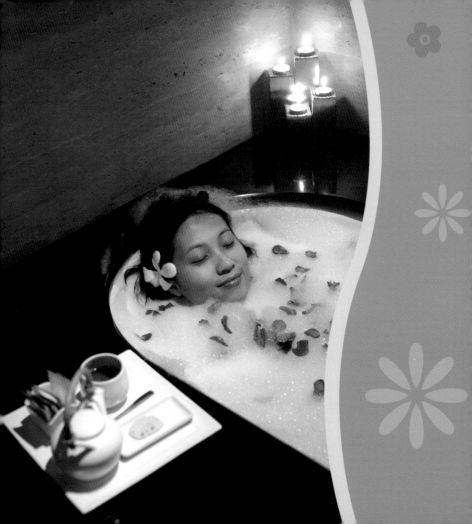

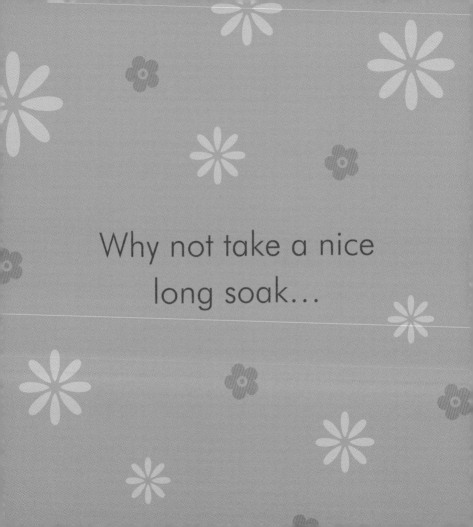

Why not take a nice
long soak…

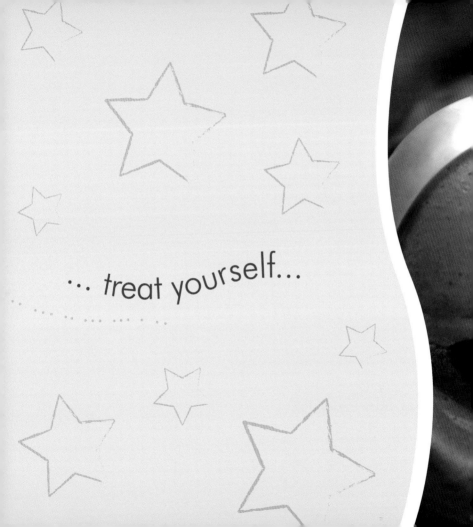

... treat yourself...

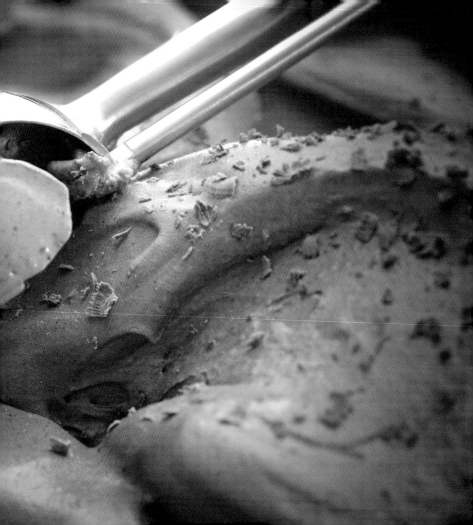

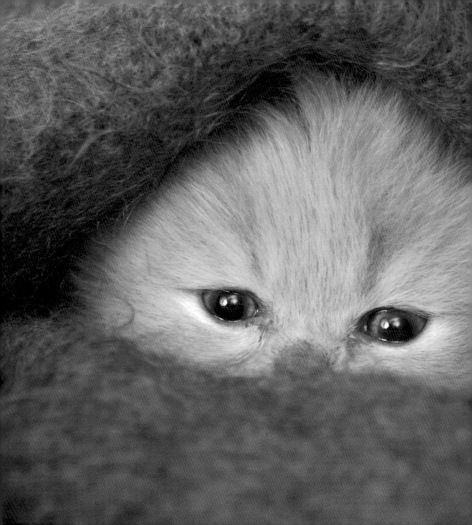

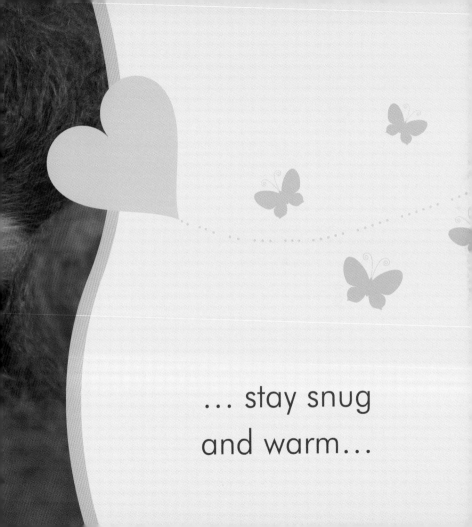

... stay snug
and warm...

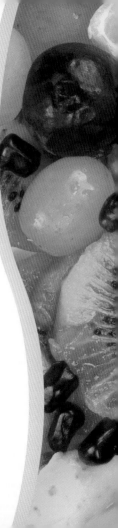

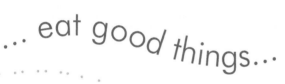

... eat good things...

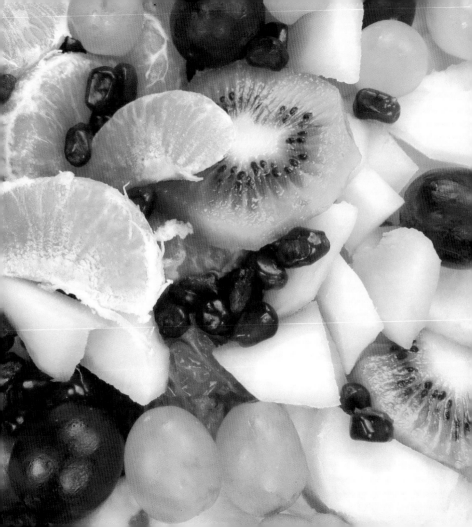

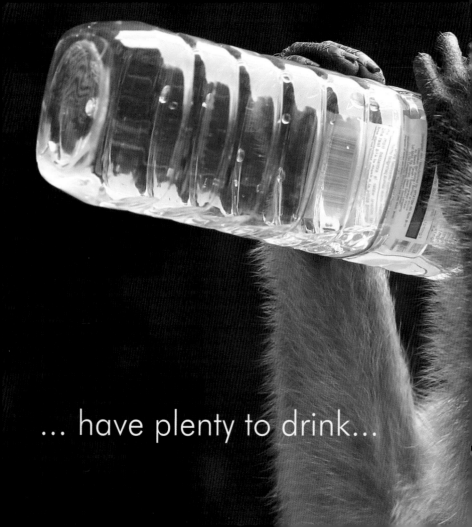

... have plenty to drink...

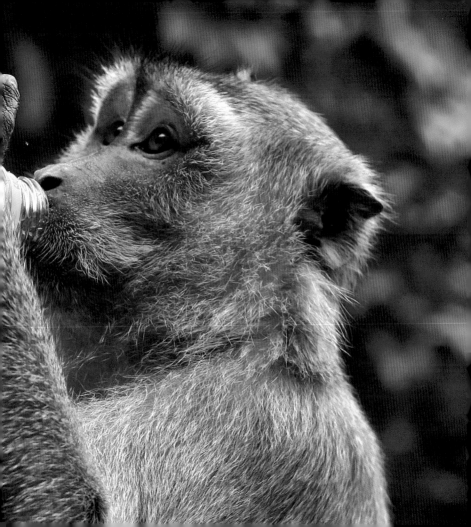

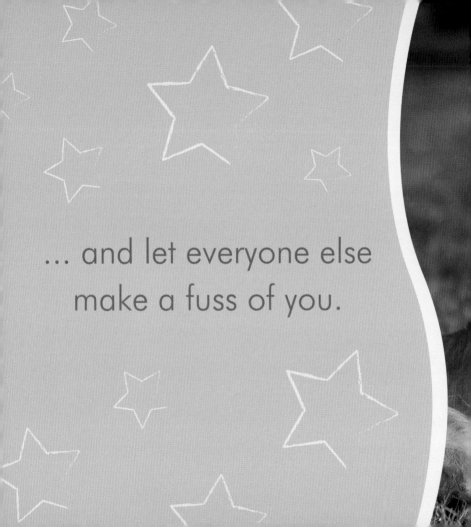

... and let everyone else
make a fuss of you.

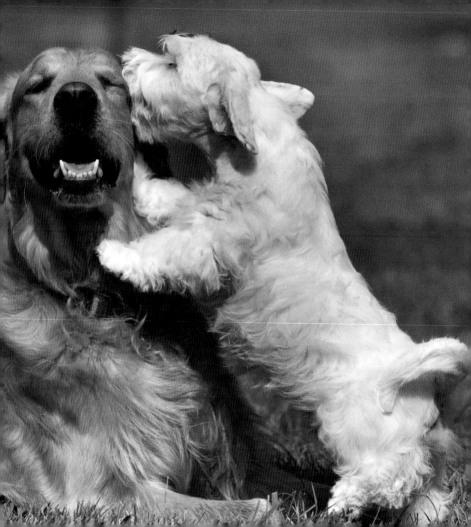

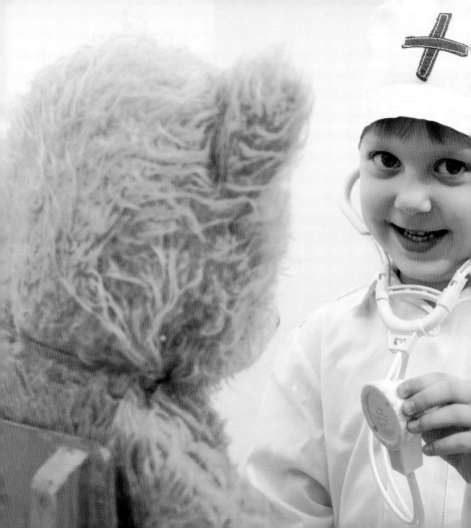

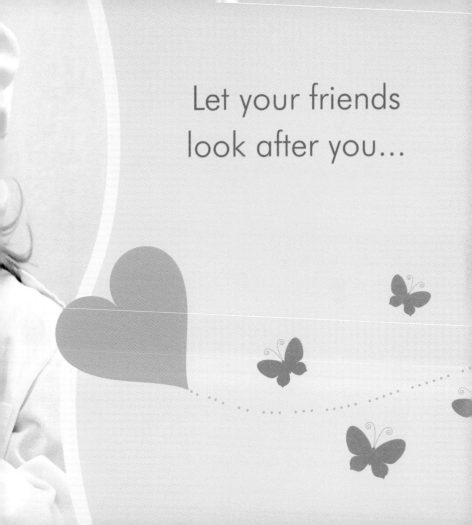

Let your friends
look after you...

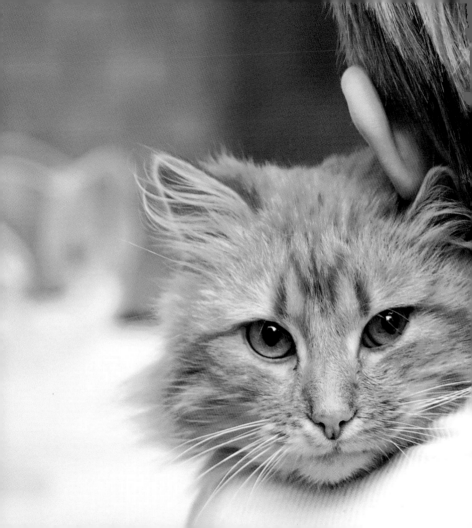

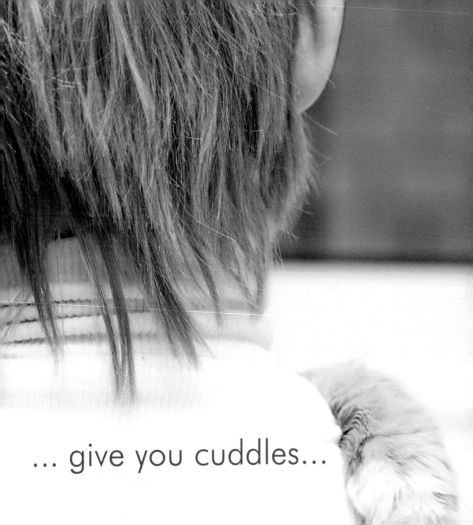

... give you cuddles...

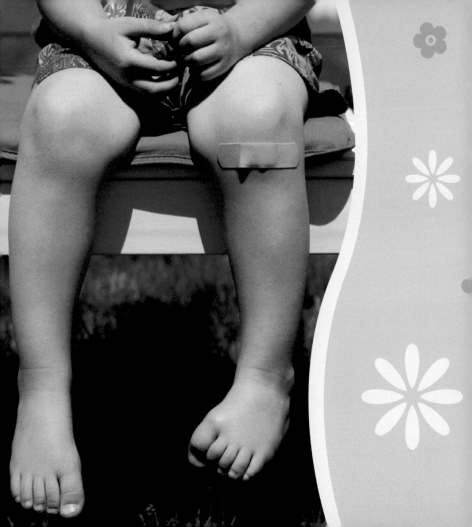

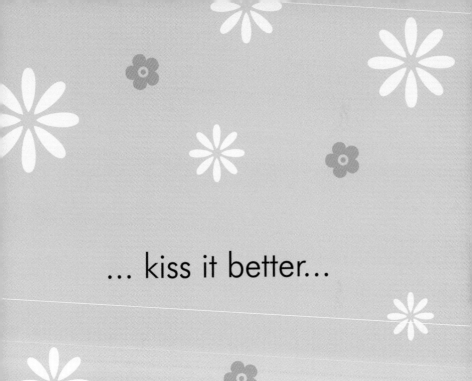

... kiss it better...

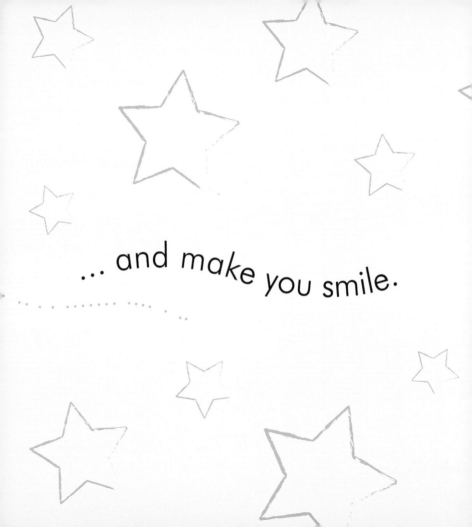

... and make you smile.

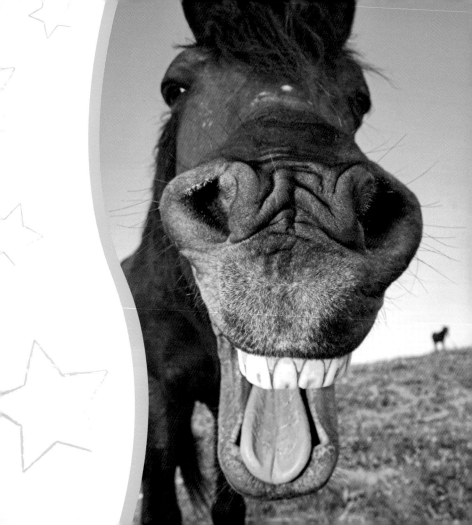

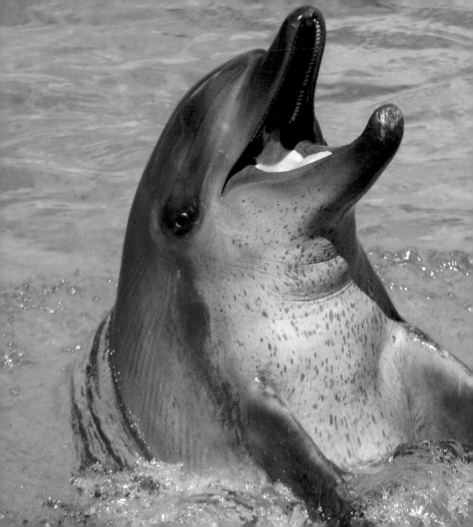

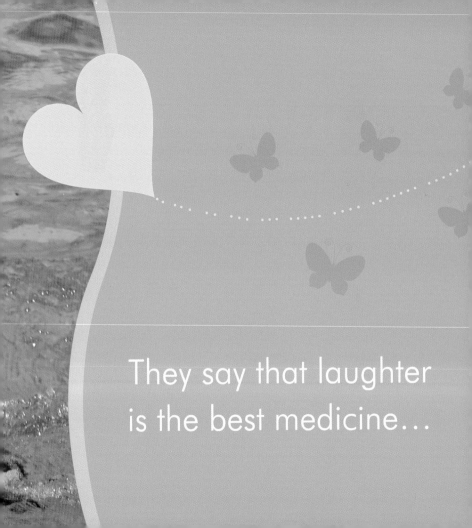

They say that laughter
is the best medicine…

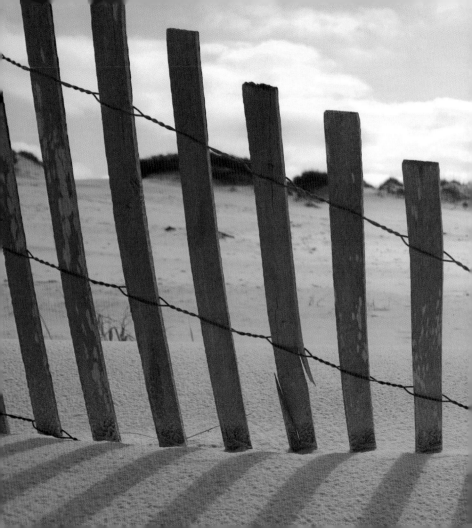

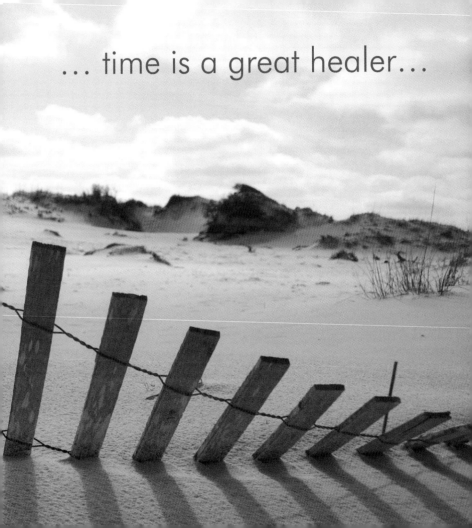
... time is a great healer...

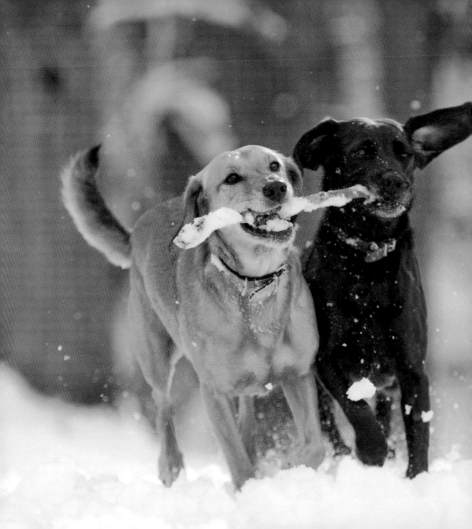

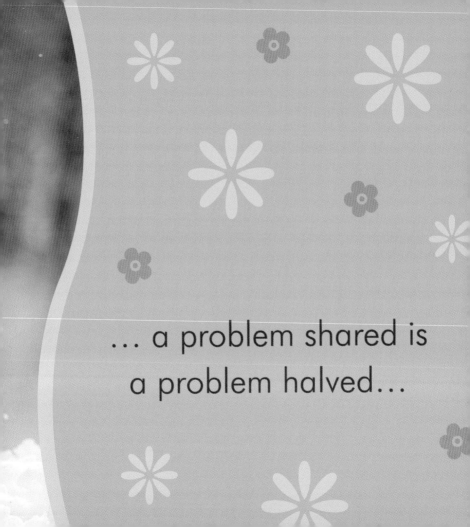

... a problem shared is
a problem halved...

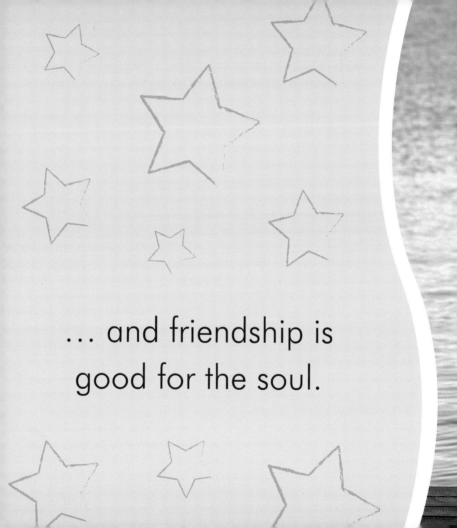

… and friendship is good for the soul.

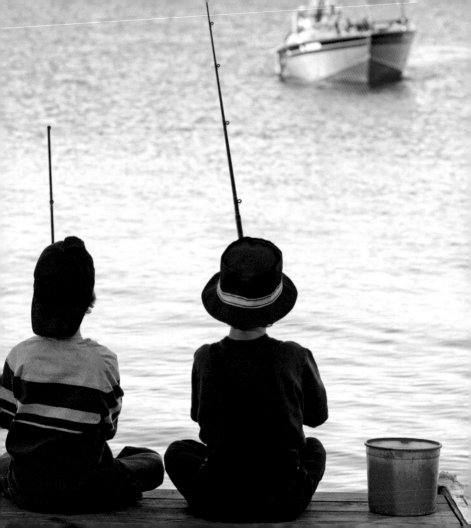

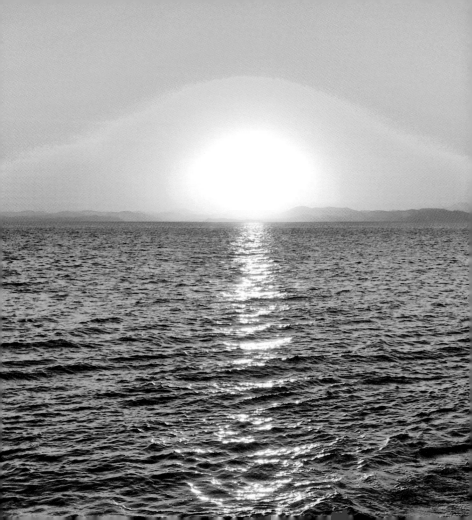

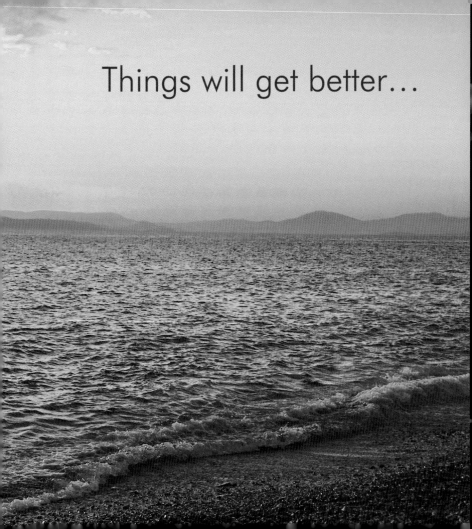

... so think positive
thoughts...

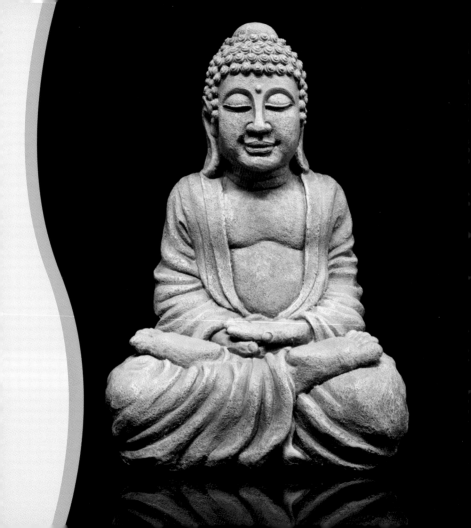

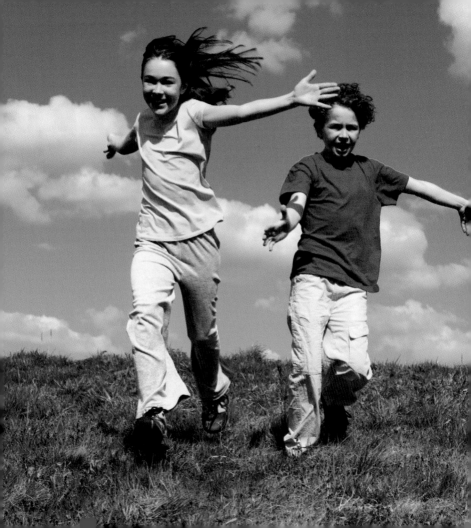

... of happier times...

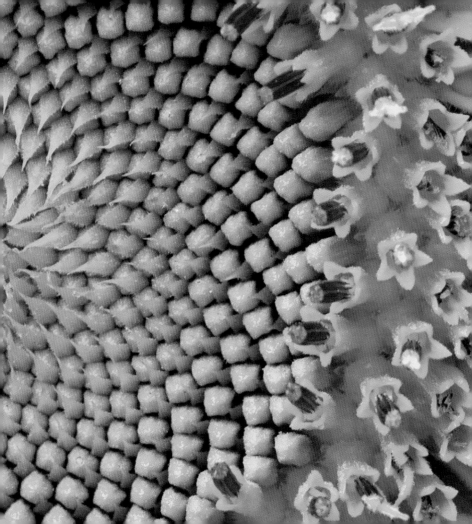

... and a bright future.

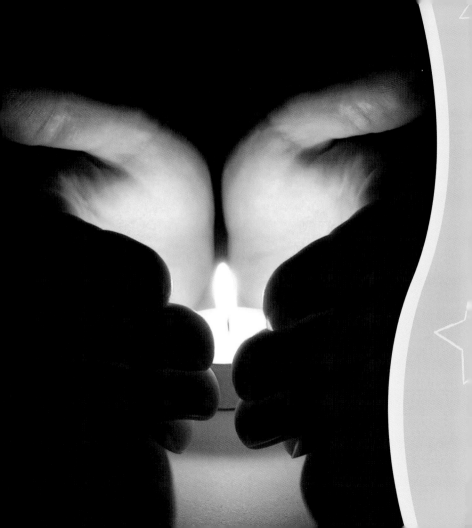

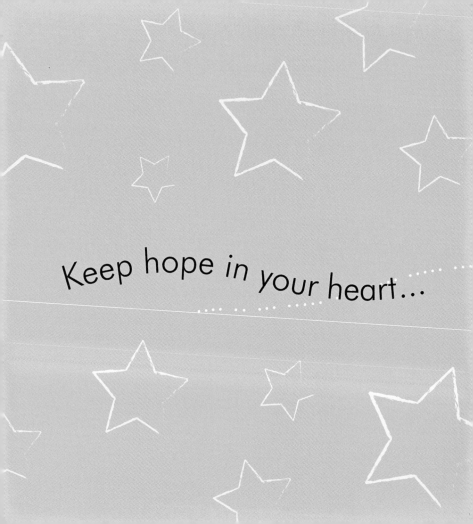

Keep hope in your heart...

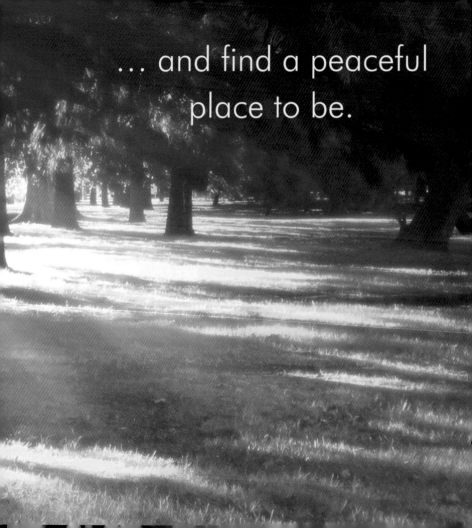

... and find a peaceful place to be.

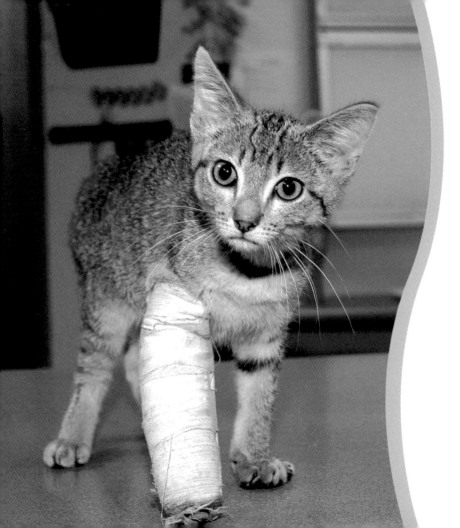

It won't be long until
you're back on your feet.

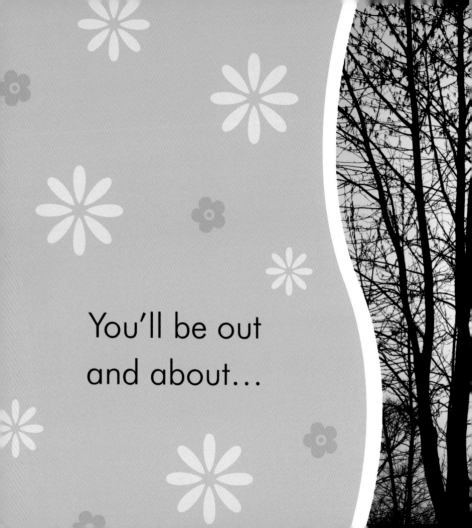

You'll be out
and about…

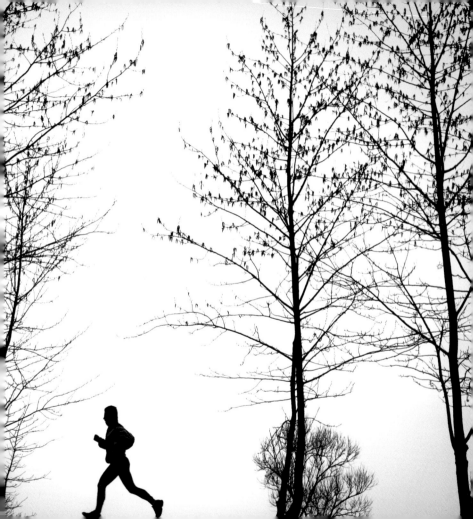

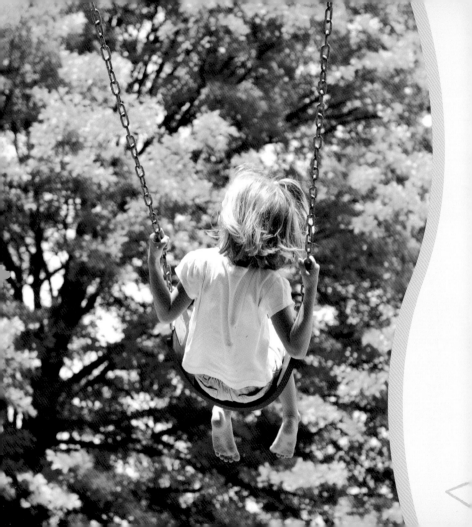

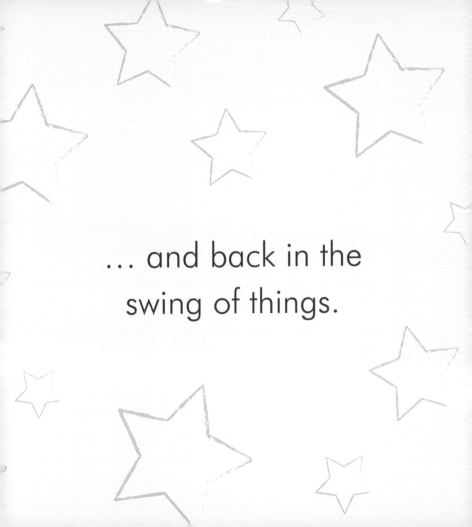

… and back in the
swing of things.

Before you know it you'll
be yourself again...

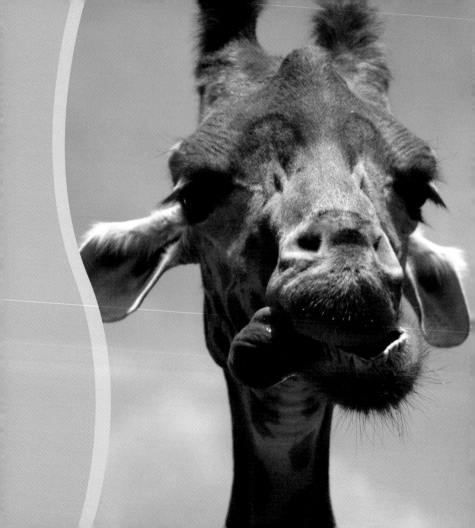

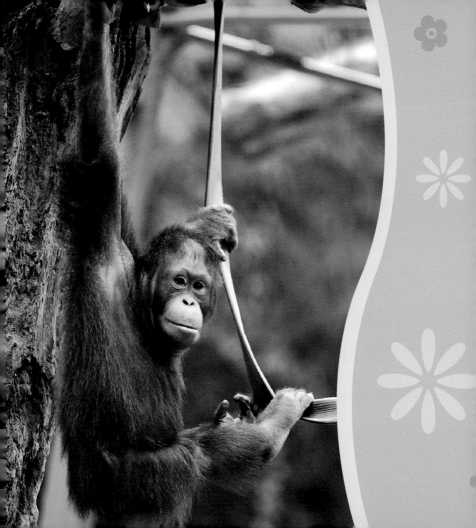

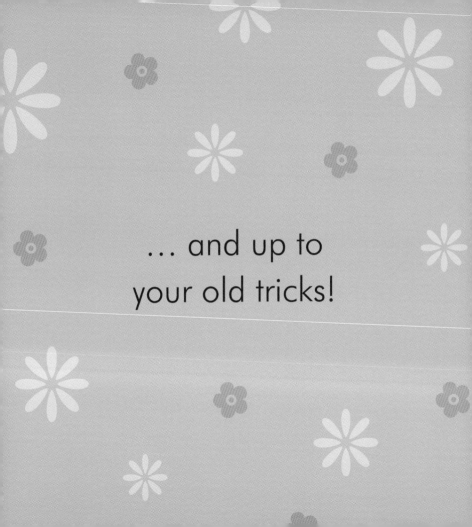

… and up to
your old tricks!

Here's to a
speedy recovery.

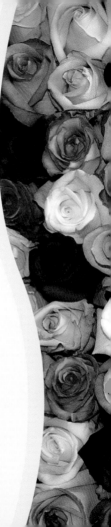

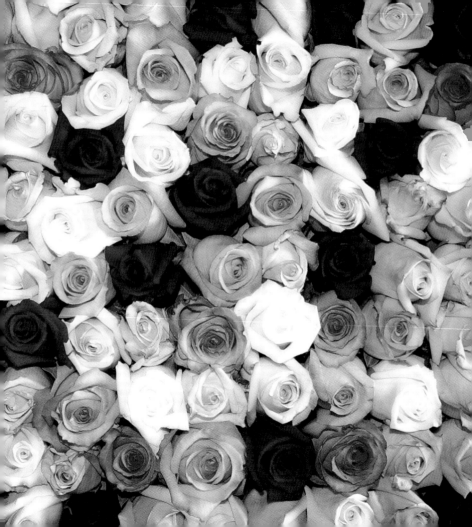

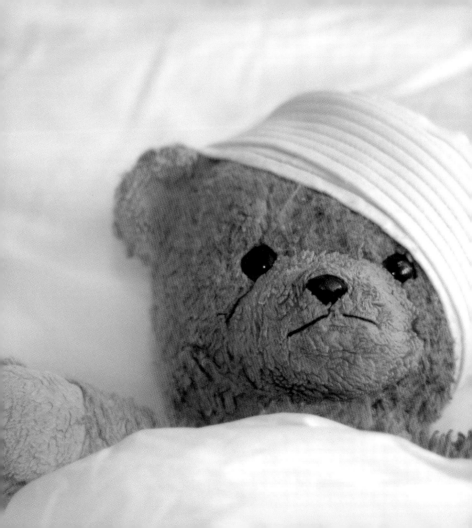

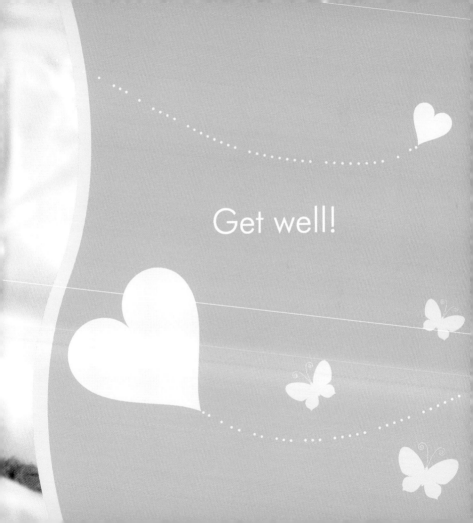

Get well!

Have you enjoyed this book? If so, why not write a review on your favourite website?

Thanks very much for buying this Summersdale book.

www.summersdale.com